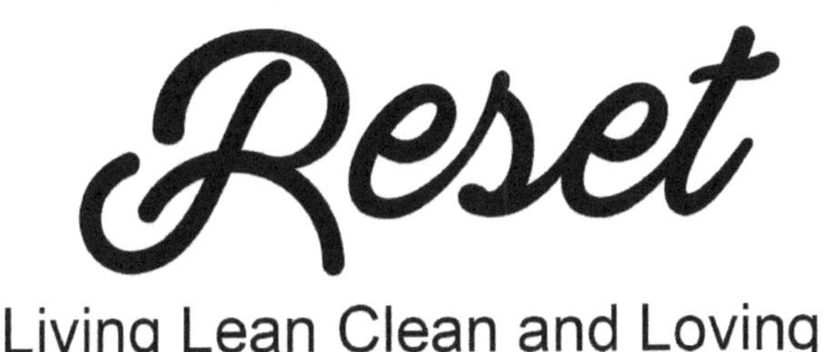

Reset

Living Lean Clean and Loving It

by Rachel Christian

Contents

For most of us, achieving weight loss and good health can be an uphill battle, often filled with frustration and disappointment, and sometimes ending in disempowerment. There are several different reasons each of us may choose to embark on this journey, but whatever the reasons, we usually go about achieving it in the same way: 'Diet and Exercise to Lose Weight.'

For those of us who have managed to achieve weight loss and subsequently better health, the feelings of confidence and renewed energy are usually accompanied by those of accomplishment, energy, vitality, ability, confidence, power, passion, renewed purpose and improved self- esteem. However we often have feelings of failure, frustration and disappointment when we are only able to achieve weight loss temporarily - or worse, unable to achieve this feat altogether.

These negative feelings are disempowering and often recur as we enter the vicious cycle of 'Diet & Exercise to Lose Weight' (DELW).

In my case, weight loss was achievable but never sustainable until my 'accidental' shift in focus. Having hit my target weight, for the first time I decided to use my sense of power and accomplishment to improve other aspects of my life. Although unintentional, I transitioned from a weight loss journey to a healthy lifestyle journey and began to experience an improved balance between what I now know as my 'Primary and Secondary Foods.'

We nourish our bodies with these. Primary Foods are often overlooked but are critical in achieving a healthy lifestyle. They can be described as those foods which feed our soul - namely Spirituality, Relationships, Career & Exercise. Our Secondary food is Nutrition - the food we eat. When our Primary Foods are balanced and satisfying, our life feeds us, and what we eat becomes Secondary.

I now coach my clients along these same principles, passed on to me through my training at the Integrative Institute for Nutrition (IIN). Instead of using the power from achieving weight loss to improve the balance between their Foods, my clients and I work together to first improve the balance, which then leads to sustainable weight loss and a consistent healthy lifestyle.

The more Primary Food we feed ourselves, the less we depend on Secondary Food. On the other hand, the more we fill ourselves with Secondary Food, the less space we leave for Primary Food - our true source of nourishment. This is why many religions and cultures practise fasting, to open channels to receive a greater amount of Primary Food.

It is my experience and observation that the greater the balance between our Primary Foods and our Secondary Foods, the easier it is to achieve permanent weight loss and subsequent health gain.

In my practice over time, I have observed that those attempting to lose weight and gain health fall into one of three categories:

1. Those who have NO balance between their Primary Foods (Spirituality, Relationships, Career, Exercise) & Secondary Foods (Nutrition)

2. Those who have a fair balance between the first three Primary Foods (Spirituality, Relationships, Career) but limited balance between Exercise and their Secondary Food.

3. Those who have a good balance between all of their Primary Foods (Spirituality, Relationships, Career and Exercise), and limited knowledge about their Secondary Foods: What should I eat and how should I be eating?

Together, my clients and I identify which category applies to them and then we proceed to establish small behavioural changes through our LeanClean Rules of Operation (LCRO), to develop habits leading to improved balance between the Foods, thus achieving sustainable Weight Loss & Health Gain.

LCRO are different for everyone. They must be achievable, so it is important that we start small and work our way up. In this Guide I have tried to mention the LCRO that are most common to all of my clients. The number of rules will vary from person to person, and all rules are NOT incorporated at once, but over time, as we progress through my 6 month programme.

It is also important to note that being accountable to me makes it is a bit easier for my clients to develop these habits. The key to your weight loss success with this Guide is holding yourself accountable, or having an accountability partner who is vested in your success.

And even prior to your starting to read this manual, a VERY important question you need to ask yourself here and now, with full and complete honesty, is:-

Do you truly believe that achieving weight loss and attaining and maintaining a healthier lifestyle is something you WANT to do or something you feel you MUST do?

WANTING to do it is fine. It means that there is a desire, a yearning to be healthier and to possibly alter your lifestyle to do so.

However, feeling that you MUST do it - for the wellbeing of yourself, your family and those around you- and to use your healthier lifestyle as the springboard for pursuing and achieving your other life goals in order to live a longer and more fulfilled life- will make all the difference in how you receive this information and how you act on it.

So are you ready for the RESET that you MUST do?

And remember as you read on from here, that you need to start small and once you are able to remain true to your first commitment or timeline, it will become easier to increase your efforts.

My goal is to help my clients be Lean and Clean from the inside out!

So here we go! The journey begins!

I was 19 years old and in quite good health when I left Jamaica to go to college. However, a couple months later I became terribly homesick and began to experience feelings of low energy, mood swings, insecurity and demotivation.

Growing up, I was always supported and encouraged by my mother who used her knowledge of God and strong spiritual foundation and faith to guide me. My parents were divorced when I was 8, and although my father played an active role in my life, I was raised by my mother. I always felt much loved by my mother, and although my sisters and I fought terribly, there was a lot of love among us as well. I did well academically and was very good at tennis which contributed to a great sense of accomplishment and esteem. My social life was very active and included many supportive friends.

Without this support system, I began using food for comfort. I would make late night runs to the corner store for chocolates and chips; I ordered pizza frequently, and cafeteria meals consisted of grilled cheese sandwiches, fried chicken, pasta, burgers and fries. I rarely had fruits or vegetables and always opted for sodas and sugary drinks instead of water. I most definitely did not work out and gained as much as 60 lbs in my freshman year. Worse were the feelings of low mood, foggy brain, lethargy, anxiety, and hopelessness. I desperately wanted to rid myself of these feelings and because I associated them with my weight gain, I began my career as a 'serial dieter'. From the "egg and coffee diet" to the "liquid diet"-- you name it, I tried it - all in an effort to lose weight and regain positive emotions. I didn't realise then that these feelings were a result of my overall health, and not directly related to my weight, so dieting was not the cure. Thus began the cycle: low feelings ->'Diet and Exercise to Lose Weight' (DELW) weight loss -> temporary feelings of empowerment ->low feelings -> food for comfort-> weight gain-> feelings of disempowerment-> 'DELW' -> weight gain, and so on.

Although I managed to experience confidence, renewed energy, accomplishment, power, renewed passion, renewed purpose and improved self- esteem when I lost weight, these feelings of empowerment were temporary and unsustainable and I would therefore start the cycle all over again. I now know that my inability to manage my weight was a result of an imbalance between my Primary and Secondary Foods.

I was able to land competitive summer internships and graduated college on time with a good GPA. However I can safely say that I was unable to maximise my potential during my college years. I did not live my best life because I was oblivious to the critical role that optimal health played in doing so.

Once I returned home, I was in my comfort zone: I began a career in a job I enjoyed- thanks to some wonderful support from my dad- I started playing tennis again and I was surrounded by my friends and family. My eating was not the best, but it was far better than it was at college, and so I enjoyed my life once more.

In 2007, I married and immediately started a family. After I gave birth to Gabrielle, my first child, I began working out and resumed my DELW regime. I managed to lose the baby weight, approximately 65 lbs, within 4 months of Gabby being born and was able to maintain my weight for about 2 years. When I think back, I realise that I was only able to manage my weight because I had a good balance between my Foods, although at the time I had no concept of Primary and Secondary Foods. I had re-established my relationship with God; I was doing well at work; I was still in wedded bliss; I had good friends, and a pretty good self- care routine. However, I still accredited my weight maintenance to my strict DELW regime!

Two years after having Gabby, Adam and Jacob were born within one year of each other and after the birth of Jacob, my youngest child, I experienced a bout of postpartum depression, similar to the low feelings I had had at college. However they were exacerbated by feelings of inadequacy as a wife and mother. I had never particularly envisioned a life of marriage and children (maybe because my parents divorced when I was 8- but more about that later), and I often wondered how I ended up here, like this. The guilt which followed these thoughts was even worse than the insecurities. "What was wrong with me? How could I be so ungrateful?"

I was on maternity leave so I was not working, but I did not have the energy to go to church and so I was unable to connect with myself on a higher level. I did not have the desire to interact with my friends or family and my marriage was not in a good place, which was a source of additional stress. At times I did not even want to get out of bed to play with my children, much less workout. And the more uncomfortable I felt in my clothes, the more junk I ate. By this time I had lost all sense of direction and drive, and was almost mentally paralysed. In other words, both my Primary and Secondary foods were out of balance.

One morning my daughter wanted to play but I was feeling such low energy that I started to cry. When I looked up, Gabby was staring at me. This was an 'aha' moment for me and I remember thinking to myself that my children deserve more than this. They needed a mother that was full of life - an energetic, passionate being, able to maximise her potential. Moreover, I thought to myself, "I am going to miss my best life ever". And so I began my 'Diet & Exercise for Weight Loss' regime once again.

As I achieved my weight loss goals, the feelings of empowerment came back and I was able to be what I wanted to be for my family. However, coming from that all-time low, paired with the fact that I had my children to consider, I worked more purposefully on other aspects of my life.

I wanted to give Gabby, Adam and Jacob the same love, encouragement and support that I received growing up. And I wanted to guide their conduct in the same way that my mother did mine, so I became more purposeful in my quest for a meaningful relationship with God. I began working again, and I quickly learnt that not every 'friend' was a good friend and embraced the art of 'loving from afar.' I also worked purposefully at improving my relationship with my husband and began to practise more self-care. The more I worked on these other areas of my life, the more effortless working out and eating properly became. In other words, the remarkable difference in how I felt actually allowed me to manage my weight more effectively.

I was so astounded by this that I became passionate about sharing it with others. I wanted everyone who faced weight management challenges similar to mine to feel as empowered as I did. I spoke with my friend and mentor Dr. Daniah Baugh @thebreathlife and she introduced me to The Institute of Integrative Nutrition (IIN). After a year-long course I became a Certified Health Coach- a supportive mentor and wellness authority working with clients to help them feel their best through food and lifestyle changes. Instead of prescribing one diet or one way of exercising, Health Coaches tailor individualised wellness programmes to meet their clients' needs.

Helping others is therapeutic for me and helps me to move further along my path to achieving a healthier lifestyle. Before we go on, I find it important to mention that I am by no means perfect, and still struggle with a few unhealthy habits myself. Like everyone else, I have good and bad days, and at times I have found it impossible to cope with my bad days. However, I believe that the most important thing is that I continue on my path of self improvement day by day!

The closer I am to me, the closer I am to Him who is within me, and the more in tune I am with my higher self is the more stable I feel - Rachel Christian

Spirituality

Several things come at us from many directions on a daily basis: balancing household matters, career, relationships etc. Our inability to adequately manage and respond to these things can leave us feeling overwhelmed, inadequate or unable. These feelings, no matter the source, adversely impact our ability to achieve our healthy lifestyle goals. In order to manage these things effectively, we have to be able to deal with them rationally. We have to be able to deal with life's situations from a clear, balanced and organised space within - what I call a Core or Spirit. The closer I am to me, and to He who is within me, the more robust my Core/Spirit is, and the less emotionally stressed I feel, because I am reacting to things rationally and not emotionally.

Studies have found that many health problems are related to stress, which seems to worsen or increase the risk of conditions including obesity, heart disease, Alzheimer's , diabetes, depression, gastrointestinal problems, and asthma. The less emotionally stressed I feel, the more able I am to consistently maintain my healthy lifestyle habits, because by improving the principles which govern my actions and reactions (aka livity), by remaining centred and strengthening my Spirit, I am nourished.

As a Christian the actions I take to develop my Spirituality are directly related to my belief in Jesus Christ. Whatever your belief, I have found the following principles are necessary for the strengthening of Spirit and I encourage my clients to incorporate them into their lifestyles.

LeanClean Rules of Operation for Spirituality

Give Thanks either each morning before rising, or at night before going off to sleep. It is as simple as thinking of three things which happened the day before or that day, and verbally expressing gratefulness for the occurrence.

That's it. Simple. Some may want to write them down, some may not. Some may have more than three things, some may have less. Whatever it is, this simple exercise helps me to feel more resilient and to think less about what I don't have.

I also practise and encourage my clients to write thank you notes if time permits, or to think about someone who has done something nice for them, and mentally thank the individual.

Research in positive psychology shows that gratitude helps us feel more positive emotions, relish good experiences, improve our health, deal with adversity, and build strong relationships. Both Harvard & UPENN health studies actually show that if you do this right before bed it increases wellbeing.

Think Abundance Whether we believe it or not, we have a choice in how we think. Thinking abundantly does not mean ignoring very real problems and disappointments. What it does mean is believing that "there is enough, that you are enough, and that the best option in life is win-win for everyone"- www.unitnet.com It means that when faced with a circumstance/situation I deliberately choose to think in abundance as illustrated by Aaron Endre below:

> Scarcity Thinking: There will never be enough;
> Abundance Thinking: There will always be more
>
> Scarcity Thinking: Compete to stay on top;
> Abundance Thinking: Collaborate to stay on top
>
> Scarcity Thinking: Hoard things from others;
> Abundance Thinking: Be generous with others
>
> Scarcity Thinking: Don't share knowledge;
> Abundance Thinking: Share knowledge
>
> Scarcity Thinking: Don't offer to help others;
> Abundance Thinking: Freely offer help to others

Scarcity Thinking: Suspicious of others;
Abundance Thinking: Trust and build rapport

Scarcity Thinking: Resent competition;
Abundance Thinking: Welcome competition

Scarcity Thinking: Afraid of being replaced;
Abundance Thinking: Strive to grow

Scarcity Thinking: Believe times are tough;
Abundance Thinking: Believe the best is yet to come

Scarcity Thinking: Believe the pie is shrinking;
Abundance Thinking: Believe the pie is growing

Scarcity Thinking: Think small and avoid risk;
Abundance Thinking: Think big and embrace risk

Scarcity Thinking: Fear change;
Abundance Thinking: Take ownership of change

Thinking abundantly helps us to live a fuller life- we feel happier, we are more generous, more creative and more inspirational and we are able to take advantage of more opportunities that come our way. When we think BIG we act BIG and so we become BIG.

Here are some examples of how I purposefully changed my way of thinking in some of the areas of my life:

1. Area/Situation: My initial weight loss and weight maintenance success. My friends began asking me for advice on what to do and how to do it.

   Old Scarcity Belief/Action: My initial thought was to hold on to my knowledge and information and not share it. I thought, "I should be the only winner." I also thought, "What if they start to look better than I do?"

   Purposeful Abundance Belief /Action: Give freely what you are able to. I shared my knowledge with my friend freely and embraced the feeling of healthy competition. I am able to achieve more when I make competition healthy, because I do not feel threatened or pressured.

2.   Area/Situation: My decision to become a certified health coach. I was apprehensive about registering for the course

Old Scarcity Belief/Action: "Who is going to pay me to coach them? I am not going to be able to make back the money that I spent to enrol in this course."

Purposeful Abundance Belief /Action: "What I have to say is powerful; I have already helped so many people and there are so many more out there that want my help."

3.   Area/Situation: Writing this Guide. I was apprehensive about writing this manual.

Old Scarcity Belief/Action: "There are so many manuals out there, is my information really relevant? Will people be interested in what I have to say? What if no one buys my manual?"

Purposeful Abundance Belief /Action: "There is enough space out there for my manual to be relevant because the pie is not shrinking, it is growing. Everyone will love what I have to offer because my experience, like everyone else's is unique. And If no one buys my manual it is ok; it is better for me to have tried and failed at my passion, than to never have tried at all! I wrote my Guide- Reset- Living Lean Clean and Loving It!"

Vision Boarding My sister Nicole @nicolemclarencampbell introduced me to this powerful tool used to help clarify, concentrate and maintain focus on specific life goals. It is a board on which you display images that represent whatever you want to be, do or have in your life.

Vision Boarding works because of the Reticular Activating System (RAS) in our brains. The RAS is the part of the brain which alerts us to new stimuli in the environment. Each time we look at our vision board, our RAS reacts to the images, dreams and power words on the board and alerts our brain to notice the images in our environment.

Love, Peace, Beauty, harmony and Joy are the things that push us to do great things, while obstacles, hindrances, and obstructions are what hold us back. Unfortunately, most of us see the physical signs of what holds us back and that can be paralysing. Placing images that represent Love, Peace, Beauty,

Harmony, Joy etc. on our Vision Board make our goals tangible and I use mine to offset physical signs of obstacles.

According to www.selfgrowth.com the general elements that a well-designed vision board should include are:

Visual. Your subconscious mind works in pictures and images, so make your vision board as visual as possible with as many pictures as you can. You can supplement your pictures with words and phrases to increase the emotional response you get from it.

Emotional. Each picture on your vision board should evoke a positive emotional response from you. The mere sight of your vision board should make you happy and fuel your passion to achieve it every time you look at it.

Strategically-placed. Your vision board should be strategically placed in a location that gives you maximum exposure to it. You need to constantly bathe your subconscious mind with its energy in order to manifest your desires quicker than you hope.

Personal. Negative feelings, self-doubt, and criticism can damage the delicate energy that your vision board emits. If you fear criticism or justification of your vision board from others, then place it in a private location so it can only be seen by yourself.

I encourage my clients to display images of their healthy lifestyle goals. I believe this moves them further along the path to attaining them

Swerve Fear Over the years I have observed that as my clients attempt lifestyle changes they are often stricken by fear, specifically the fear of failure. Some are so afraid of failure, that they even undermine their own efforts through procrastination and not following through with the actions necessary to achieve their goals. This fear is often accompanied by anxiety, which can also prevent goal achievement because it is when we are relaxed that our mind becomes clearer, we feel more in control and we are better able to focus on the actions necessary to achieve our healthy lifestyle goals.

Although I still experience fear at times, I am better able to push through it by doing the following actions which I encourage my clients to do, to quell anxiety:

Use Inspirational Words Inspiration and assurance bring us relaxation. My main source of Inspiration are the words contained in the Bible which assures me that fear is not what God gave me, rather it is an emotion designed to hold me down. Whatever your source for inspiration, assurance and peace, keep them on top of your mind, readily available for use when needed. Memorise words of Inspiration, assurance and peace. I encourage my clients to write them down and stick them on the mirror, in the car, on the laptop, and on the fridge.

Command Your Day Commanding the day to day actions necessary for achieving my goals is a powerful tool for actualising visions and has an impact on me being able to carry them out. I am aware that to live my healthiest life now, each day I need to be at peace, to manage fear, nervousness or anxiety. I need knowledge, wisdom and understanding, as well as energy and vitality, to be able to guide those around me and complete my tasks efficiently. Some may command their day using scripture, while others use regular words. Some may command 3 things while others may choose to command 10. Here is an example of how I command each day:

"In the name of Jesus I declare that I am blessed and highly favoured, I declare that my household is blessed and highly favoured. I declare that no weapon formed against me or my household shall prosper. I declare that my youth is renewed like the eagles and that I will run and not grow weary, I will walk and not faint. I have peace which surpasses all man's understanding. Through wisdom my house is built, by understanding it is established and by knowledge the rooms are filled with precious and pleasant riches. Though weeping may endure today, I know that Joy cometh in the morning and today is a joyful day. Thank you Father that I am the head and not the tail, I am above and never beneath. Thank you Father that I do not have a spirit of fear but of power, love and a sound mind. My household is blessed with health, strength and long life"

We all face unique situations in life. Think about the actions necessary for your desired outcome and be purposeful in commanding them! For instance, let's say you are nervous or anxious about a presentation: think about what you need to be feeling to alleviate those emotions- peace, strength, power, knowledge, wisdom, and understanding. Command those attributes. If you have an argument with someone, and you still feel as if it is unresolved, you may feel anxious, jealous, worried, or angry. The feelings you want to experience here are peace, joy, love, forgiveness. Command those.

Remember: your word is your power! Think about how you want things to unfold and command that outcome.

Worship with people of like mind. Whether weekly, bi-weekly, monthly or bi monthly, I have found that there is real power to be had from worship with others, which I believe energises the intimate time spent connecting with my inner self. "The time spent drawing inward and focusing your energy on clearing your thoughts leads to a drastic reduction in stress levels. After spending time in the place of worship, you feel lighter, more confident and free from worldly worries." - healthfitnessrevolution.com

Participating in praise and worship with others is very effective in strengthening of Spirit, and so church attendance has recently become a consistent part of my lifestyle. However, consistency was not possible until I found a church with which I could connect. The fact that my sister-friend Latoya @latoyaamoy attends the same church makes it all the more interesting as we are able to share our thoughts and feelings and encourage each other.

Remember, "church" is a group of believers and not a building and so we must be mindful of the fact that it is very possible to go through the motions of regular worship without wholesomely benefitting.

Of course adherence to these rules does not happen overnight but instead over a period of time, and they become less of a rule and more of a habit through consistency, focus and discipline. Start small and be patient with yourself!

Relationships are two-fold - the relationship we have with ourselves and the relationships we have with others.

RELATIONSHIP WITH SELF

I do not believe that life just happens to us- we are not innocent bystanders. I believe that we happen to life. "Life is experienced through us, not outside of us. Our perception of ourselves has a significant impact in determining the experiences that we have in life. Simply put, the more we love ourselves, the easier life will be because we will be better equipped to achieve the goals we have set for ourselves."- www.huffingtonpost.com

Having a good relationship with myself provides a basis for remaining consistent on the journey toward better health, including weight management, as this creates the desire within me to want the best for myself. The happier I became with who I was, the more my emotions shifted from working out and eating clean because I did not like my body - to exercising and eating clean because I enjoyed working out and experiencing the elevated energy that comes from eating well.

I am by no means totally in love with myself - this is still a work in progress for me. But I am better than I was yesterday, and I will be even better tomorrow.

Being happy with ourselves does not come overnight and initially, daily practice is important to shift our mindset. To start, we should consider what we are doing to support ourselves. This will be different for everyone. For example, if you are an introvert, you may want to think along the lines of "How am I renewing and recharging myself?" If you are an extrovert, are your social connections feeding you? If you are somewhere in the middle, then you want to be thinking along both lines. You and your body are miracles and you are to be celebrated!

In addition to incorporating some of these rules into my life, I encourage my clients to do the same and together we come up with:-

LeanClean Rules of Operation for My Relationship with Me

Honouring Your Word: Most of us strive to keep our word but often fail, sometimes due to circumstances beyond our control. Over time this causes us to become lax with our word and we stop making an effort. When we break our word, it lowers our self-respect and self-trust, and the power of our word becomes diluted- we no longer believe in our power to proclaim something as true, and see it manifest in our lives,

"Each time we keep our word, we create something in our lives because our word creates a certain amount of energy that is used in manifesting our reality. So, when you state something, you are already half-way there. When you stop honouring your word, the energy becomes jammed and gets blocked. The result is that fewer things manifest for you, and fewer people (especially you!) believe in your power to create. Therefore, it is crucial that you pay close attention to each word you say, and each promise you make." (Margot Zaher).

Our word is literally our power, as it fuels our actions, and our actions accomplish our goals. For instance, when I promise myself to work out and I do not, I feel disempowered about working out and it is easy to miss day 2 and day 3 and day 4, and before I know it, I've missed a month. This leads to disempowerment in other areas of life - a deadline at work, or a commitment to a friend. The same thing can happen with my eating clean efforts: when I eat something that I have promised myself I wouldn't, it disempowers me, and so it becomes easier for one bad meal to turn into two and two into three until before I know it, I am right back at square one; feeling more incapable than ever before.

Affirmation & Talking Yourself "Up": Positive affirmation and self-talk help to quiet our biggest critic- our inner critic. BUT in order for affirmations and self- talk to work, they must be totally honest and true! For instance, instead of saying "I can handle this new project" say "I am scared about handling this big, new project, but I am learning to have confidence in my ability to achieve my goals." When we script our affirmations and self-talk with honesty, then the statements aren't "empty self-praise" or temporary "mood-boosters." They are honest, self-respecting assessments about where we are at, what we are learning, and what we are capable of becoming. They are affirmations of truth—and the truth will set us free.

Get Sleep: If you are feeling run-down, struggling to focus, or are feeling irritable for no clear reason, you may want to look into your sleep patterns. Maintaining an adequate amount of quality sleep is essential to your optimal health and well-being.

In his article entitled "Why You Gain Weight by NOT Sleeping, How to Sleep Away the Pounds", Dr. Adam J. Rubenstein, MD writes that, "Accumulating research shows that getting good quality sleep is essential for your waistline, and if you have been missing out on sleep even by an hour or two, it could be making you fat," suggesting that there is a possible link between sleep loss and disrupted levels of appetite-regulating hormones, causing bouts of overeating to result in weight gain.

Adequate sleep may be more difficult for some than it is for others, but the key is to start somewhere. My clients usually start with two nights a week, doing whatever it takes on those two nights to ensure that they are in bed, 'Lights out,' by 9 or 10pm ensuring 7-8 hours of sleep.

I really struggled after getting home from a long day at work, when my kids would draw my evening out all the way until it was my bedtime. This was driving me crazy. Not only did I not have any time for me, but I was also exhausted when I had to 'rise and grind' and get it done all over again the very next day. I had to take the painful decision to ensure that, no matter what, my kids were in their own beds by 7:30 pm. This literally changed my world. Was it hard at first? YES! However I pushed through until it became a habit for them to be in bed by 7:30, and for me to be in bed by 9:30pm. It was well worth it as now I wake up feeling more rested on a regular basis.

Based on Dr. Rubenstein's recommendations, here are some tips for when getting adequate sleep is an issue:

- Stay away from stimulants like caffeine, nicotine and alcohol, before bedtime. Although alcohol initially induces sleep, it eventually produces stimulating effects after a few hours, causing you to wake up often, which negatively affects the quality of sleep.

- Turn off the TV, draw the blinds, and ensure your bedroom is a sleep-inducing environment. This is especially important if you work night shifts, as light is a powerful signal to your brain that it is time to wake up.

- Turn the alarm clock away from you or put it at least 3 feet away so you resist the urge to check the time.

- Don't eat dinner too late as this may cause indigestion and insomnia. If you need to snack close to bedtime, make it a light snack like almonds, yogurt or raisins. CHEW SLOWLY AND WELL!

- Keep your bedtime the same, in order to regulate your sleep cycle. If you want to change your bedtime to an earlier time, do it in small 15-minute increments, to allow your body to adjust.

- Resist the "itis". Resist drowsiness right after dinner by doing mildly stimulating activities: choose an outfit for the next day, call a friend, clean up the kitchen, pack or prep for the next day etc. If you give into the "itis" chances are you will wake in the middle of the night and have difficulty falling asleep.

Do Not Compare Yourself with Others: Comparison is the thief of joy. My good friend and happiness coach Rochelle @rochellegapere is a huge advocate of this. It is natural to compare yourself with others, however constantly doing so on a regular basis can create feelings of envy. In addition, it can lead to becoming obsessed with where you fall short. Envy and inadequacy can leave you feeling paralyzed. Strive to compete with yourself, ensuring that you are in a better place than you were yesterday.

Avoid Gossip: Negative thought processes, upsetting discoveries, and the expression of anger can be the results of gossiping. It is used to elevate our sense of self above that of another person. To be honest, I used to get a real kick out of hearing the latest gossip. However, entertaining as it may be, gossip has destructive powers. The closer I got to myself, the more aware I became that using my word to destroy others did not arouse authentic positive emotions within me. In fact it aroused inauthentic, negative emotions having the power to block my blessings. And so now, as much as I can, I avoid gossiping. Remember, our words have power and when we use our words destructively, it tampers with the energy that surrounds us. It slows us down.

Self-Care: "Some self-care measures may seem like luxuries, but they are actually essential for your health and well-being. When we become familiar with our needs and honour them, then our energy is boundless and our potential is limitless." - IIN. For me, this may be as simple as a 7:30 bedtime rule for my kids, to occasionally sending them to their grandparents. Whether it be treating myself to a spa visit or making time to laugh with my friends or dating my husband, self-care is the foundation of a satisfying, full life and it gives me the energy that I need to exercise.

Here are some other examples of things I put into place to ensure my self-care:

- Whenever my hair is intact I feel intact, almost like I have nitro in my engine. I feel a bit more confident and able. The hairdresser takes time and can be pricey and my workout usually leaves my hair 'blah'. I decided early on that my hair would not be an excuse for me not to work out and so I found a workout-friendly hairstyle, and I also started practicing to do my own hair in between hairdresser visits. I bought a soft cap steamer and a small flat iron that I could handle. When I had hair, I could even roller set!

Whether Birthday, Mother's Day, or Christmas I opt for Spa gift certificates from friends and family, when they ask. I stack them in what I call a "care" jar and whenever that day comes along where I feel I can't go on anymore, I draw for my "care" jar. I also buy and use facial masks, or Google 'homemade facial masks.' Think about the things which make you feel alive. Write them down and think of ways you can put them into place to ensure that those things happen.

RELATIONSHIP WITH OTHERS

Maintaining good relationships with others makes life more fulfilling; on the other hand, bad relationships usually inflict emotional stress, which negatively impact our health. In addition to incorporating some of these rules into my life, I encourage my clients to do the same and together we come up with:-

LeanClean Rules of Operation for My Relationship with Others

Move Wide: When it comes to family, friendships and romantic relationships, the transfer of energy is real. If we are constantly surrounded by, interacting with, having sex with, or pouring our feelings and ourselves into an empty person then eventually they will suck us dry. Sometimes our closest friends, because of their own issues, will try to put us down in an effort to make themselves feel better. They may do this sarcastically to our face, or worse, they may talk about us behind our back.

It is okay to distance ourselves from these people, to love them from a distance. The more I hung out with people that made me feel bad about myself, was the more disempowered I felt. On the other hand, the more I hung out with people that motivated me and encouraged me, the more able I felt.

Here are some other actions that I encourage my clients to take in an effort to improve their relationships with others:-

Listen more and try to talk less

React to others with less emotion

Compliment often

Judge less

Practice feelings of abundance

Avoid gossip

Be kind

Forgive Easily: Let's elaborate on this, because many of my clients suffer a lot of pain because of this. They hold on to grudges, malice, and are unable to practice forgiveness. It might be instinctive to want to meet hurtful behaviour with more hurtful behaviour, but all it does is create more pain, and that's not what you want. It is in your best interest to quickly put an end to the hurt and move your awareness, attitude, actions, and life into a positive, effective state. Be the strong one in the interaction, in the relationship. Be the one who acts with positive power. By doing this, you will free the energy and space necessary to follow through on the action needed to achieve your healthy lifestyle goals.

We spend a huge chunk of our day working and so it is very important that our work space is filled with positive emotions and good energy, or at the very least, that it is not filled with negative emotions and bad energy. Eight hours of toxic energy each day is equal to 40 toxic hours a week and 40 toxic hours a week is equal to 1,200 toxic hours a month, which is 14,400 toxic hours a year. Toxicity directly impacts our health in a negative way.

A lot of my clients come to me with very negative and even toxic feelings connected to where they spend most of their days- their work environment.

Firstly, it is important that we know with certainty that just because we may not be where we want to be now, doesn't mean that we will never get there. Secondly and most vital, in the meantime we must make the absolute best of where we are now in order to create the space for "where we want to be", to exist.

These are a few of the things that I did to improve how I felt about my career, which enabled me to make space for something which gives me life - Health Coaching. I encourage my clients to do the same and together we come up with their,

LeanClean Rules of Operation for My Career

Financial Health Rule: Money is the physical representation of our input at work. It's the reward we get for the hours we put in each week. I've found that a big part of our negative emotions towards our jobs has to do with money or lack thereof. How many times have we thought to ourselves, "every day I wake up at X o'clock and spend all of my time and energy doing Y, and at the end of the day I don't even have enough money to do Z."

Usually these thoughts leave us feeling inadequate, incapable, hopeless and disempowered. Undoubtedly, this debilitates us and chances are we won't be able to honour the commitments made to our healthy lifestyle change.

Oftentimes we have more financial power than we think. I, myself, used the services of a financial coach- Stephan Byam @tooltimestef and it made a big difference in my financial health. I encourage my clients to spend and save their income more wisely, by strict budgeting and/or seeking advice from a financial coach. It was an issue for me, so I met with a financial coach for one session. It was very helpful in shifting my perspective, where my income was concerned.

Organisation: According to a study in the Personality and Social Psychology Bulletin, those who felt their homes were "cluttered" or full of "unfinished projects" were more depressed, fatigued, and had higher levels of the stress hormone cortisol than those who felt their homes were "restful" and "restorative".

Another study in the Psychological Science Journal found that people who worked in a neat space for 10 minutes were twice as likely to choose an apple over a chocolate bar, as those who worked in a messy office for the same amount of time. Clutter stresses the brain and can leave us feeling overwhelmed and confused at work i.e. brain stress. And when the brain is stressed we are much more likely to resort to food for comfort.

I wasn't always good at organising my space, but luckily I have a friend Yolande @yolicess, who is the Queen of organisation! A lot of her tips have really changed my life. Here are some of those that I use and also suggest in coaching my clients:

- Try to get to work and/or any other event at least 15 minutes before the official start time. Ever heard the saying, "Early birds catch the most worms?" It is true that when we arrive early we have a chance to unwind and relax in the environment, making our minds more peaceful and better ready for the day.

- Have a to do list (I love ticking off things completed)

- Organise my workstation each evening. Clutter leaves me feeling overwhelmed and confused at work .

- Set phone alarms as reminders to complete tasks, especially those my husband asks of me. Those are really important!

- Set up schedules for each of my children at the beginning of the term to be mindful of PE days, Sports days, School meetings, holidays, homework days etc. As soon as they get a school project, I make a note of it, as well as the due date. This way nothing pops up unexpectedly.

- Make grocery lists - I absolutely dislike going to the supermarket, and the only thing that annoys me more is forgetting an item and having to go back more than once a week!

- Teach my kids how to pick up after and organise themselves, so that I do not have to do it (it takes work but they will eventually get it!)

- Set up bill payment schedules on a calendar, so that I do not forget.

- Keep my closet as clutter-free as possible.

- Organise my gym bag the night before and put it by the front door.

- Create a 'bucket list' for my life which is also on my vision board. This gives me things to look forward to, and also reminds me of achievements to feel good about.

Improving my spirituality and relationships helped to create a space for me to envision what could fulfil me career-wise, and being organised and financially healthy helped me to actualise it. The happier I became in that 8 hour chunk of my day, is the easier it became for me to do what it takes to achieve my healthy lifestyle goals.

Unfortunately there is no one magic workout that will transform your body, and there is no magic pill that I can recommend you take in order to keep you consistent in this area.

Rather, it is my experience and observation that the better the balance among the other three primary foods mentioned before, the more you will begin to embrace exercise, which will result in consistency. The less stressed and tired I am, the easier it is for me to go workout.

Exercise for me used to have everything to do with not wanting to be overweight, and so I processed exercise as going to war with my body. I used to view exercise as a necessary evil that needed to be endured -as more of a punishment- only doing it after overeating or letting myself go through the holidays or after a bad vacation. As such, my emotions and feelings easily influenced my ability to exercise and even when I did drag myself to the gym I felt more drained than anything else, making it impossible for exercise to become a consistent habit.

It is only when I shifted my view on exercise that I was able to embrace it. In addition to aiding and abetting weight loss maintenance, motion creates emotion and has the power to move us into a positive state, a more constructive or a more creative place. "Working out and exercising is the easiest way to reconnect with yourself and feel inspired and motivated again!"- Joe Duncan

As one of my inspirations @marcusricefit so rightly put it, "Now I view exercise as something I was created to do. Our bodies were created to move, jump, push, pull, lift, and be strong and powerful. Exercise is a conduit for all these things, a conduit for constantly conquering challenges, growing and thriving. It is a means to celebrate what we can do and become, and not to punish ourselves for the mistakes we make." Now, for me exercise means:

1. A boost in happiness levels, maybe not immediately, but surely overtime

2. Reduced risk of heart disease naturally

3.   Better Sleep

4.   Energy boosts

5.   Increased strength and flexibility

6.   Realised Power in achieving a daily workout goal

7.   Improved memory

8.   Increased self-confidence

9.   Better performance at work

10.   Less susceptibility to disease

11.   Longer Life

Apart from a better balance between my Primary Food groups which created a space for me to be able to shift my mental focus and view, the tool I have found most effective in developing and sustaining my exercise routine is setting rules for myself and how I operate. I encourage my clients to develop rules as well, and together we come up with our:-

LeanClean Rules of Operation for Exercise

Organisation I encourage my clients to identify ways in which they can organise to make working out as seamless as possible.

- Set multiple workout alarms, especially for the mornings. I set 6…all 2 minutes apart. By the time the 6th alarm goes off, I'm up from snoozing the 5 times before.

- Pack gym bags from the night before .

- Pack shower bags from the night before. Putting shower bags in the trunk the night before prevents the dreaded 'lugging a million bags' in the morning.

- Download series or music on phone for cardio. This can give us something else to look forward to, especially if it is a juicy series .

- Buy gym wear that you love and will want to put on. This can be expensive and so I usually hit the sales racks of quality exercise-wear for 'tun-up' deals.

Learn to Run I encourage all of my clients to join a run club, as running only requires sneakers, shorts and a t shirt.

I never considered myself a runner. I always admired runners and wanted to get into it, but it was something that intimidated me. Because it intimidated me, I made fun of it – I used to say "I'm not running unless someone is chasing me!" I only made fun of it because I thought I could not do it. But I read that running was one of the most efficient ways to lose weight and so I boldly joined a run club.

When I initially consult with my clients and ask them what they do for weight-loss cardio, most of them tell me that they walk. Although walking may be good for circulation, walking alone will not get you efficient weight loss results in good time.

In order to achieve their weight loss goals, I encourage my clients to ramp up their efforts, because nothing is more frustrating than losing weight at a turtle-like pace. Most people give up before they can realise any real results.

As mentioned, running can be very intimidating at first. The first time I tried to run I could only run for about a minute at a time. This was frustrating, but instead of allowing it to disempower me, I used this frustration to challenge myself- I would walk for a minute and then run for a minute. I would do this for the entire 5k until I could walk 2 minutes and run 2, then 3 minutes and run 3. The more I increased my running minutes, the less number of minutes I needed to walk. All this, until I was running a full 5k.

I encourage all of my clients to start their running journey like this! And then we set a goal for them to enter and complete a 5k run. Not only does it encourage consistency, but at the end of the 5k you are more running-empowered than ever before, and usually keep entering.

Workout Frequency Initially when I was trying to lose weight I worked out four to five days a week, I ran 2-3 days a week and HIIT (High- Intensity Interval Workout Training) for 30 minutes on the cardio machine 2 days a week, followed by 45 minutes of weight training. Now, to maintain, I do a 10 minute HIIT routine on the treadmill followed by a 45 minute weight training session 3 times a week. I try to include a fourth day for outdoor running. If I find that I want to shed a pound or two, I increase my workout frequency to 4 days a week, and I ramp up my outdoor running to 3 days a week. For my treadmill cardio, I increase my HIIT workout to 30 minutes. For my weight loss clients, we begin our routine by working out 4 days a week.

I work with my clients to develop their own workout frequency but this rule is mainly dependent on their weight loss goal.

Workout Time: What time of day is best for you in achieving your workout goal? What time of day will enable you to honour your workout word? That is the time of day when you are less likely to find an excuse.

When I first started my journey, I worked out in the evenings, I was never a 'morning workout person' and I cringed at the thought of leaving my warm cosy bed to go 'buss a sweat'. But then I realised that this choice was not effective in helping me to achieve my workout goals. I would pack my gym bag, throw it in the trunk and go to my office. And most times, by 3pm I had a dozen excuses (some valid, some not so valid) as to why I could not workout. I was getting to the gym on average twice a week when my goal was four times a week.

Something had to give. So I changed my workout time to the morning. This was really very hard for me at first, and of course I fell off the wagon a couple times. However, once I got the hang of it I was back on target for achieving my goal. Now, I mostly go to the gym first thing in the morning. For the most part my husband understands that working out is a part of my lifestyle, however there are times that I do have to compromise my morning workout- times when an "iron tight grip" prevents me from getting out of bed at the crack of dawn!

Some of my clients very well achieve their workout goal in the evening. In any case, selecting the right time of day for our workout is a major key to making exercise a habit.

Most of my clients live overseas where climate change is an issue and so waking up early to go to the gym is just not an option, especially where they rely on public transportation. Where this is the case, I recommend that my clients download or purchase any of the following CD's to workout at home:

- "T 25 with Shaun T"

- Winsor Pilates

- Beach Body Fitness Programs

- Kamp Kamila 10lb pledge

Incidentally, Kamila @iamkamilamcdonald is also my friend and an inspiration to me. In addition to this, I recommend that my overseas clients join franchise gyms which have several different locations. This way, they are able to take advantage of locations which may be close to home and close to work.

Calorie Burn: I do not believe in calorie counting as a regular part of a healthy lifestyle, but using a heart rate monitor to track calories is a huge motivational tool that I utilise in coaching through the initial stages. For my clients who are trying to lose weight, our rule is 350-500 calories of cardio before weightlifting. This can usually be achieved best with a 5k run, an hour-long spinning class, or a treadmill or elliptical HIIT workout.

Weight Training: In all my efforts throughout the years to transform my body, I never actually saw mind blowing results until I began to weight train. I encourage my clients to begin weight training because:

(a) It sculpts and transforms the entire shape of the body achieving a well-toned physique.

(b) It burns fat at a much faster rate

(c) It leaves us feeling mentally empowered

Contrary to popular belief, weight training does not have to result in big muscles and bulkiness, or in women "looking like a man". Weight lifting results will depend on how heavy we are lifting and how we are eating.

As beneficial as weight training is, it can be intimidating to walk into a gym with all of those machines. Sometimes we just don't know where to start. Personal Trainers can be costly, and so where this is an issue for my clients I ask them to work with a trainer for 3 sessions to learn proper form and weight to lift. Form is essential to achieving desired weight training results.

Protein Shakes: I encourage my clients to drink protein shakes because they help to build muscle which helps to burn fat at a faster rate. If weight loss is the goal, I advise my clients to select protein shakes with less than 2 grams of sugar.

Workout on Vacation: When I used to see other people on vacation, at breakfast and walking around, in workout clothes I used to think to myself "Wow, some vacation!" I never thought I would be one of those people. Now I do not leave home without my workout clothes. I carry my workout clothes on vacation and as a part of my programme, my clients must do this as well. Before the vacation begins, we decide how many days we will work out and what those days are.

Not only does working out on vacation give me the energy that I need to vacation well, it also keeps me on track with how well I eat on vacation.

Accountability Partners: I try to surround myself with good workout influences as much as possible. In doing so, I am motivated to Just Do It. Luckily, my friends work out as well, but I also ensure that I flood my social media with workout fanatics and physiques that I admire like:

> @nicole_mejia
> @getfitandthick
> @juliejigsaw
> @babymommafit
> @iamkamilamcdonald

As well as motivational pages like:

> @afrogirlfitness
> @weightlossfatloss
> @weightlossadvice
> @trainandtransform

Track Your Progress: Tracking your progress by recording your weight and measurements can be a huge motivational tool in the initial stages of your journey. The further along you go, tracking becomes less and less frequent until your clothes more or less become your tracking tool.

These rules may seem like a lot at first, and like anything else will take some getting used to. In time, the behaviour resulting from these rules becomes second nature and will require little thought or effort.

Once we are able to incorporate these small behavioural changes into our daily lives, we can achieve more of a balance with our Primary Foods. This balance will make it easier to nourish ourselves properly with the food we eat.

GET STARTED WITH EXERCISE!

1. I believe in Bio individuality- what is for the goose is not necessarily for the gander and so I do not believe in setting a specific program to address the needs of several different people.

    Initially you want to be clear and specific about your goals and intentions for yourself regarding your Healthy Lifestyle. Once identified, create your Healthy Lifestyle Vision Board.

2. Using both the Measurement Guide and Weight/Measurement Chart provided at www.leancleanreset.com record your initial weight and measurements. Measure and weight yourself every 2 weeks. As time goes by and you get closer to your goal, you can start to record monthly until it does not feel necessary to record at all. I used to do this, now I do not weigh and measure at all, instead I now use my clothes as a guide.

3. Workout- Cardio & Weight Training

    Workout at least four (4) days a week. A standard workout should include both Cardio and Weight Training.

    (a) Cardio can be either of the following:

    1 hour spinning class

    - Run Club

    - Outdoor Running/ Run Club

    - 40 of Minutes of HIIT on the treadmill or elliptical

Whatever you choose to do, you should aim for a minimum calorie burn of 300- 500 calories and remember a Polar watch is more accurate than cardio machine calorie readings.

If you opt for a HIIT workout, you may use the Lean Clean HIIT Workout Guide provided at www.leancleanreset.com

    (b) Weight Training

of the four days, designate a day for each of the following:

- Legs

- Chest & Back & Abs

- Arms & Shoulders & Abs

- Abs

Feel free to use my weight training guide available at
www.leancleanreset.com

4. Check your heart rate monitor watch and aim for initial calorie burn target of 600-750 per gym session

5. Drink protein shake within half hour after workout

"If you take care of yourself by feeding yourself beautiful food, you're much more likely to engage in actions which nourish your soul such as exercise, prayer and word meditation, and other techniques that make your life rich and vibrant. When you feel great, you're able to move through your days with joy and ease, creating and nurturing supportive relationships and a career you love." - IIN

There are hundreds of diets, meal plans, meal options and recipes available online that can help us to lose weight, so it's obviously not just lack of knowledge that prevents us from managing our weight and achieving weight loss. Many of us fail to remain in control of what we put in our mouths, because there is a deficit in our Primary Foods.

Before attempting to discuss healthy eating with my clients, I talk about the effects of food on our bodies in an effort to have them begin to think about food differently.

The food that we eat is absorbed into our blood down to a cellular level and changes the shape and very function of our cells. It also alters how chemicals and hormones behave in our brain. Undoubtedly, food is directly related to how we look, but more importantly, it is related to how we feel, how we think and how we behave.

Food is information that has the power to heal or harm our immune system as it imprints our cells with information. When we eat healthy food our cells work properly. When we eat unhealthy food we experience poor cellular function that can damage the body, such as inflammation (the root of all disease). In addition, the chemicals, additives and toxins contained in food, change cell function.

Once I share this type of information with my clients, the "Food for Weight loss" concept gradually shifts to the "Food for Health" way of thinking, and this creates the environment for transformation.

Although how we look can be a big motivator in achieving weight loss and healthy lifestyle change, it is how we feel that is responsible for keeping us consistent and pushing us through the journey of lifestyle change.

When I began fuelling myself with the best foods I began to not only experience weight loss, but I also experienced feelings of increased energy, vitality, clarity, and I was better able to focus. In experiencing these feelings, I was more motivated to eat these foods and better able to remain consistent in my clean eating efforts - thus maintaining my weight.

While discussing Secondary foods, we must rely on our knowledge of Primary Foods. The more we know about Primary Foods, the easier it is to see why we eat for emotional reasons, and why we binge eat. When we are depressed or experiencing low self-esteem – we are starving for Primary Food. No matter how much Secondary Food we eat, we will never feel satisfied. The need for love, power, or mere acknowledgement, drives the desire for excess secondary food.

Bearing in mind that food directly impacts our energy, it is important to know about the Energetics of Food. Traditional Chinese Medicine (TCM) focuses on using food to prevent and treat disease. Instead of describing foods by how much protein, fat, or calories they contain, TCM focuses on the quality of the food. All foods have distinct energy and characteristic properties that either make us healthy - balancing and nourishing our bodies - or create imbalances that result in sickness. This is food energetics. This knowledge can help build a stronger sense of health and well-being by eating foods that have a different impact. Like the saying goes, "You are what you eat." Check out the Food Energetics guide at www.leancleanreset.com

It is also important to mention that we absorb more of the nutrients from our food when we are mindful of our food when we are eating, slowing the pace of our meals and eating in a relaxed setting. In addition to this, eating from our own garden or buying our produce from the local farmers' market will leave us feeling more connected to our home or local community. The body is more in touch with the natural order of things when we eat seasonally and locally, and we are then able to maintain balance from the inside out.

I encourage my clients to eat less meat, milk, sugar, and 'chemicalised' artificial junk food. I also recommend less coffee and alcohol. Less does not mean none, it just means LESS!

We first examine what their current eating patterns are and what foods they like to eat. Once this is established, we move towards creating healthier versions of these foods- we tweak the way they are prepared and the portion size.

- Preparation.

  - Coconut oil replaces vegetable oil and a very, very limited amount is used in preparing the meals.

  - Baking, grilling, steaming or broiling are the methods to use instead of frying or stewing meat and fish.

  - We do not use sauces or ketchup, nor do we have gravy with our meals.

- Portion Size

  - For portion size guidance, check out the Lean Clean portion guide at www.leancleanreset.com

Again, as with my Primary Food Groups, the tool I have found most effective in developing and sustaining habits are setting rules for myself and how I operate. I encourage my clients to develop rules as well, hence our:-

LeanClean Rules for How We Eat.

Swapping Out: I encourage Swap Outs. We swap out white foods (sugar, flour, pasta, rice, bread, and pastries and other standard desserts containing white sugar) for healthier unrefined options. Here are some of the Swap Outs that I encourage my clients to make:

- Juices & Sodas For Water: I drink 3 litres of water a day. Why? Water circulates between cells and inside organs supplying nutrients and excreting waste. This has cleared up my skin, which now has a healthy glow. Water keeps you "Fuller for Longer", by hydrating your body, because when your body is dehydrated you tend to crave more. When I craved, I craved more SUGAR! Understanding what sugar does to your body is, in and of itself, motivation to make this shift.

At first, drinking so much water can be difficult for my clients. I find that it is easier for me to get my 3 litres in when:

- I consciously avoid taking small sips of water at a time, instead I drink a significant amount of water at one time. This allows me to achieve my water goal at a faster rate

- Drink room temperature water, if for no other reason but that it allows me to drink more at any one time.

Remember, it is not about dieting, it is a lifestyle shift!

Sugar wreaks havoc on the blood sugar level. First, it pushes it sky-high—causing excitability, nervous tension and hyperactivity, and then it drops it extremely low—causing fatigue, depression, weariness and exhaustion. I refuse to carry out any part of my day feeling like that ON PURPOSE. To stop eating sugar is not as easy as it sounds. Quitting suddenly will cause withdrawal symptoms such as headaches, mood swings, cravings and fatigue.

I encourage you to take a look at the "Common Foods with the Highest Amounts Of Sugar" illustration available at www.leancleanreset.com

Again, the more we are able to achieve balance among our Primary foods, the easier it is for us to achieve our Secondary food goal.

In order to reduce sugar cravings, I:

- Eat sweet vegetables and fruit (portion consciously)

- Get more sleep, rest, and relaxation. If you are in a chronic state of stress and/or sleep deprivation, your body will crave the quickest form of energy there is - sugar

- Get physically active. Being active helps balance blood sugar levels, boosts energy, and reduces tension, which will eliminate the need to self-medicate with sugar!

Here are some other swap outs which I recommend my clients do gradually, within the first three months of my program:

- Brown rice instead of white rice

- Quinoa instead of rice

- Cauliflower rice instead of rice

- Sweet potato instead of rice

- Fish instead of meat (on some days)

- Beans instead of meat (on some days)

- Salads instead of carbohydrates and starches (on some days)

- homemade dressings instead of store bought salad dressings (www. leancleanreset.com)

- Sauces and condiments with reduced sugar instead of regular ones

Meal Prepping & Meal Guides: When I first began my journey I meal prepped religiously on a weekly basis. I learned very early on that not having the right food on hand at all times could derail my efforts. Being prepared and organised with meals in your initial stages of this journey will prove critical to developing proper eating habits.

When I did not have a healthy meal on hand, one of two things happened-

- I would not eat -triggering a fleet of emotions including resenting my journey.

I would be easily irritated and agitated; feel stressed out and have headaches. Worst of all, I would eventually stop at the first fast food restaurant I could find, using starvation as an excuse.

- I would eat crappy food. This speaks for itself.

The first excuse I had where meal prep was concerned was, "I do not have the time." However, after much consideration, and trying to do this food thing every other way, I realised that meal prep was the only thing that could help me. So, I made the time. My first attempts were shaky to say the least, but as time went by I improved. I encourage my clients to get started like this:

i. Buy Meal Prep Containers and a lunch kit

ii. Choose a day of the week when you will meal prep. Ensure that it is a day when you have time for yourself. I actually use my meal prep days as a self-care tool.

iii. Create a Grocery List. This will keep you organised, and you will spend less time in the supermarket.

iv. Buy produce at the market. It will be more economical and you will feel more connected to your home and local community

v.   Pick recipes that make Meal Prep easy. I do not choose elaborate recipes because the process is designed to prepare and store food for up to 3 days at a time. The more elaborate the recipe, chances are having been stored for so long, the meal won't taste good.

vi. Keep it simple by prepping a basic carb or starch to go with a protein option, or a basic protein to go with a carbohydrate or starch option.

vii. Create a Meal Guide. Bio Individuality - there is no perfect way of eating that works for everybody. Bio-Individuality means there is no "one-size-fits-all" diet. Each person is unique with highly individualised nutritional requirements. Differences in anatomy, metabolism, body composition and cell structure influence your overall health, and the foods that make you feel your best - or as I like to say: "What fatten hen kill dog."

In coaching my clients to lose weight, I do not give them specific Meal Plans per se. Instead, I teach them how to balance their foods, and we work together to incorporate meals they like.

Remember, there are endless meal plans available on the web for free, and any one of them, if followed correctly will more than likely give you your desired result. However, I have observed that blindly following a "one size fits all" meal plan does not lend itself to lifestyle change.

For this section I would like you to get four coloured highlighters orange, blue, green and pink

1. Highlight the following foods Orange. These are examples of meal options which have a higher content of starch & carbs than the other meal options discussed:

BREAKFAST OPTIONS

1-2 cups Tuna & Cabbage, 2 slices Sweet Potato, 1 Green Banana

1 Slice whole Grain Toast with Peanut Butter & 2 boiled egg whites

1-2 cups Sardine, 2 slices Sweet Potato, 1 Green Banana

1-2 cups Callaloo & Saltfish, 2 slices Sweet Potato, 1 Green Banana

1-2 cups Saltfish, 2 slices Sweet Potato, 1 Green Banana

3 Pancakes, Watermelon

1-2 cups Overnight Oats Parfait

1-2 cups Maple Nut Granola

1-2 cups Chia Seed Pudding

2 Banana Nut Oats Muffins, watermelon

1-2 cups All Bran Cereal (Whole Foods)

1 cup Oatmeal with ½ banana, almonds, raisins

LUNCH/DINNER OPTIONS

3-4oz Meat; Vegetables; 1 small Sweet Potato or 2 Green Bananas

2-2.5 Cups Ravioli Vegetable Soup

2 cups Korean Beef Stir Fry

3-4 oz Fish; Vegetables; 2 slices Sweet Potato or 1 Green Banana

3-4 oz Seafood; Vegetables; 2 slices Sweet Potato or 1 Green Banana

Fried Brown Rice, Salad

2. Highlight the following foods Green. These are examples of meal options which have a higher content of protein & vegetables than the other meal options discussed:

BREAKFAST OPTIONS

Boiled Egg Whites & Turkey Bacon

3 Scrambled Egg Whites & Melon

3-4 Egg White Vegetable Omelette

2 cups Parfait

Codfish & Cabbage, 2 slices sweet potato

Tuna & Cabbage

Smoothie

Fruit Plate

2-3 Egg Muffins, Cantaloupe

Green Juice & Fruit

LUNCH/DINNER OPTIONS

Tuna Salad and Salad or Steamed vegetable

Squash & Tofu Curry Salad or Steamed vegetable

Stuffed Peppers with Cauliflower Rice and Salad or Steamed vegetable

Pureed Vegetable Soup with Tossed Salad

Citrus Pan Seared Fish with Cauliflower Rice and Salad or Steamed vegetable

3-4oz Protein with Salad or Steamed vegetable and Corn

3. Highlight the following foods Yellow. These are examples of lighter snack options than the other snack options discussed:

SNACK OPTIONS

1-2 Cups Fruit: Watermelon, Cantaloupe, Apple or Berries

1 Hard Boiled Egg with Salsa

Chia Jelly & Apple Slices

Green Juice

1 Cup Tuna Salad

2 Cups Soup

Carrots & Avocado Dip

Carrots & Low Fat Hummus

1- 2 Cups Sorbet

1 Corn on the Cob

4. Highlight the following foods Pink. These are examples of heavier snack options than the other snack options discussed:

SNACK OPTIONS

Cucumber Slices with Peanut Butter

3 slices low sodium deli meat & 2 pieces melba

Tuna Salad & Melba

Chocolate Popsicle

1 Tablespoon Dark Chocolate Chips

1 Banana Nut Oats Muffin

2 Oatmeal Cookies

2 Slices Melba Toast with Chia Jelly or Avocado Dip or Peanut Butter

For the most part, I encourage my clients to eat more protein and vegetables, hence your meal guide should look more green than anything else. I also encourage them to eat their heaviest meal first and we generally try to eat 2 ½ -3 hours apart. Green Juice should also be a part of your initial meal plan, start with one day a week and increase to three. One ingredient green juice is usually easiest and so where time and clean-up are an issue, I encourage my clients to start with cucumber or celery juice.

Firstly, I ask my clients to choose a day of the week when they would like to have a meal or snack that is not in line with our goal, kind of like a "free meal." In doing this we discuss the fact that a free meal is not the same thing as a "free DAY" and we agree that it will be pencilled in only ONCE a week. Once they identify this day of the week, we pencil into one meal or snack slot on our table, which is basically divided into 6 eating times per day over a 7 day period as follows- Meal 1-Breakfast, Meal 2- Snack, Meal 3- Lunch, Meal 4-Snack, Meal 5-Dinner, Meal 6-Snack. You do not have to eat six times a day, snacking is optional.

Once we pencil in our 'free meal,' we go about pencilling in our breakfast options. I ascertain from our discussion what day they feel like they will want a heavier breakfast. I opt for an orange breakfast on Monday and in most instances, so do my clients. I also ensure that the days I work out heaviest, like run days or leg days are on the same days as orange breakfast days. We then proceed to pencil in our orange breakfast option and we do an orange breakfast every other day for 4 days. Pencil in all other breakfast slots green.

Once our breakfasts are pencilled in we move to lunch. Most of our lunches pencilled in are green- except for Saturday which is usually reserved for errands on the road and dining out with friends- and so my clients usually opt to pencil in orange lunches on this day. To make space for "Sunday Dinner" discussed below, we usually pencil in a green lunch on Sundays.

Now on to dinner. As with lunch, most of our dinners are also green options, except for Saturday, which is orange. The other exception is Sunday, which is culturally known as 'Sunday dinner,' time spent with family around the dinner table. Bearing culture in mind, I encourage my clients to eat out of the family pot if so desired, hence an orange dinner on this day. While 'eating out of the pot' on a Sunday, I encourage that they replace rice and peas with salad and if unable to do so that they opt for brown rice or limit white rice and peas to only ½ cup.

Balancing snacks is also simple, On weekdays where we have orange break-fasts, we pencil in two yellow snacks and one pink snack. On weekdays where we have green breakfast options, we pencil in two pink snacks and one yellow. On Saturday and Sunday we go for all yellow snacks.

So, it's time to level-up! Let's draw up our meal guides to include the colour coded meal options which appeal to us the most! I have illustrated a meal plan template and sample meal plan for reference at www.leancleanreset.com

Looking Up & Making a Personal Collection of Recipes: If "clean"food is unsatisfying, bland and boring, then chances are we won't turn these dietary changes into lifelong habits. In order to keep healthy food exciting, I flood my social media with healthy food recipe pages. This gives me lots of ideas and keeps things interesting. I also test recipes that I have googled. Some pass, some fail - I keep the passes and toss the fails.

As tasty as some recipes are, chances are that in the initial stages of your transition, clean eating will not satisfy you in the same way as your previous choices did. That's because you are accustomed to foods high in sugar, trans-fats, chemicals and additives that are designed specifically to stimulate and tantalise taste buds, ignoring the health aspect.

Most big food companies incorporate high amounts of sugar, additives, chemicals and preservatives in processed and packaged foods to keep us coming back for more, thus increasing their bottom line- profit. Take comfort in knowing that as time goes by, your taste buds will adjust to your new way of life and eating healthy will eventually become yummy and exciting.

Remember, discipline will play a key role here, but it becomes easier as the balance increases in the Primary foods. All this may seem very overwhelming but believe me, over time, as it becomes a habit it will become a part of your lifestyle and will become more effortless overtime so stick with it! I have provided some of my favourite recipes for the foods mentioned above at www.leancleanreset.com

TIPS FOR EATING OUT

Social interactions and entertainment often involve food. Sometimes bad food happens to good people. In order to minimise the impact of eating out with friends, I:

    i. Always try to recommend a restaurant that I know has healthy options.

   ii. Scan the menu for the healthiest options- e.g. If the soup is cream of something, I leave it out.

  iii. Am not shy. Sometimes I ask the waiter to have the chef replace my rice or potatoes with steamed vegetables or a salad.

iv. Order dessert, eat a mouthful (my indulgence!) and give the rest away; or I share one piece of dessert with friends.

v. Ask the waiter to split the meal in half, if servings are large. Or, I eat a portion and take the rest home. Sometimes a friend will be willing to split a meal with me.

vi. Always drink 2 full glasses of water before I start to eat

Incorporating Juices: Juicing is a controversial subject in the nutrition world, and juice fasts and cleanses are currently a popular dietary trend. Advocates for juicing claim it's a fast and convenient way to get nutrients into our bodies, while opponents argue that we miss out on important health benefits from the nutrient-rich skin and fibre that is extracted during the processing. Regardless of your juicing stance, a glass of your favourite greens is still a better choice than a processed, sugar-laden snack.

I encourage my clients to introduce juicing by having them identify 2 days out of the week when they will be able to juice. Usually by the end of our 6 month program, my clients are juicing 3 to 5 times a week, on average. The key is to start small. Start with easy, one-ingredient Juices such as Cucumber Juice with ginger and lime (my favourite), Celery Juice, or Kale Juice (use a small amount of pineapple to sweeten).

What's the difference between Juicing & Blending?

"A juicer will extract the juice and remove the pulp from your produce. What you're left with is all of the liquid from your veggies and fruit, and none of the pulp. A blender takes the whole veggies and fruit and pulverizes it into a thick drink. You get all of the liquid AND the pulp from your produce." www.rebootwithjoe.com

I personally prefer to juice my greens because of the more liquid consistency which makes it easier to drink. If you have a similar preference but only have a blender then a great investment would be a cloth strainer. A cloth strainer is a very fine meshed cloth that is used to filter liquids and will make blended green juice easier to drink.

As mentioned, if time and clean-up are an issue, I recommend "One Vegetable" juicing as opposed to juicing several different vegetables. My favourite "One Vegetable" juices are Cucumber and Celery.

I recommend Juicing for my clients who are trying to lose weight, since it allows you to reduce your daily caloric intake while flooding your body with the necessary vitamins and minerals. Please visit www.leancleanreset.com for some of my favourite juicing recipes.

Eat whole foods every 3-4 hours This stabilises the blood sugar. Waiting too long between meals can lead to brain fog and a crash in energy (which will make you more likely to reach for sugar, fat, or caffeine, to keep your energy up).

Keep a snack on hand at all times I keep one in my car and another in my desk drawer at all times. This way if I am running behind on my meal time, I have something on hand, reducing the chance that I may give into an unhealthy choice out of desperation. Almonds, Melba toast, KIND Bars, Popcorn, are examples of a few healthy snacks I keep on hand. Also, be sure to portion these snacks out to avoid over indulging, which can also sabotage weight loss efforts.

Say "no" to deprivation I sometimes crave the 'junk' and allow myself an indulgence so as not to feel deprived – which is no way to feel. An indulgence should be guilt free, not a binge or emotional. Again, a better balance within our Primary Food groups helps us to avoid this. If you really feel for something, have a piece of it and give the rest away.

Get the entire household involved If you have ever attempted lifestyle change then you know that it can be difficult when the rest of your household is not on the same page. In order to make my transition easier, I had to make some small adjustments where my household was concerned. For instance, I introduced my family to "Meatless Mondays," I stopped buying juice and sodas and replaced them with water and natural juices. I also introduced my family to smoothies and green juices. My children now snack on a lot of fruit and less packaged snacks and I found that getting my children involved in the preparation of healthy juices, snacks or treats makes them eager to try them out.

Chapter 7 CONCLUSION

I read a review in Forbes Magazine awhile back that examines the Qualities that High Achievers possess in common- a list that would include, by the way, a number of hugely famous, ordinary people who have done some truly extraordinary things.

It stated that :-

- Achievers believe in themselves and in their abilities

- They are positive thinkers

- Achievers recognize and acknowledge their strengths and their talents.

- They take action.

- Achievers have a sense of purpose and have an understanding of the meaning of life.

- They do what is required to reach their goals.

- Achievers recognise that if someone else can achieve something, then so can they.

The piece stayed with me a long time, and at first I couldn't quite figure out why.

But then I began to reflect on my own journey- from that little 8 year old girl whose world was shaken by her parents' separation, to the teenager who travelled abroad for college and gained so much weight as she struggled to adapt to life overseas, to the college graduate who returned home and started a career, marriage and family, experienced myriad challenges and then- in a determined effort to be a better wife and mother- RESET her life and her entire approach to better eating, better health and her overall better being.

And this is what occurred to me:-

EVERY ONE of us is uniquely capable of being a High Achiever in our own sphere. What we must do is to acquire the qualities of these other High Achievers. We too MUST experience the feelings that they do, the feelings that make it possible for these qualities to exist. The ONLY effective way to do this is through attaining OPTIMAL HEALTH. In other words, you must be feeling energetic, focused, capable, confident, secure and strong in order to have a strong sense of self, be passionate, organised, powerful and purposeful. You will then have clarity, be driven and experience your abundance. All these feelings are prerequisites for the aforementioned qualities of those who have achieved so much and who we aspire to emulate.

So as I continue to improve the balance between my Primary and Secondary foods, not only have I been able to achieve my goals, but I have also been able to achieve them at a faster rate. I have been able to achieve things that I never imagined or thought possible, including creating this guide. And as I get closer to Optimal Health, I have become more in tune with myself, which has enabled me to give more of myself to my husband and my children.

It is not possible to give OF your best if you are not AT your best. And I am now able to have a much more positive influence on my children as a result of the changes that I made. They are happier, more confident and outgoing, and better able to focus on their academics as well as their extracurricular activities. Even at their tender ages, they are also identifying goals and reaching for their dreams.

My husband has also benefited from my healthy lifestyle journey, and overall, our relationship has improved as well. I believe I have become a much better partner. This brings me back to a point I mentioned earlier in the very first chapter of this manual, about a darker period when things were not as good between us. As I look back now, with hindsight I am able to appreciate how much the divorce of my parents at such an impressionable age affected me. The truth is that like many of my peers and perhaps many of yours as well, I grew up and went into my own marriage believing that a happy union would be the perfect panacea for all my own insecurities and self-doubts, many of them harboured since childhood. I thought that falling in love and getting married automatically meant happily ever after. God knows I WANTED it to.

What I failed to realise is that no matter what the movies may say, another person can COMPLEMENT us - but they can't COMPLETE us. I also hugely underestimated how challenging it was to have to face the same person, day after and day, merging lives and all your habits- good and bad -under one roof and in one household. And becoming a mother so soon into my marriage created another new dynamic altogether, because before the two people who started that journey could fully learn to accommodate each other, there was now a third party (albeit a stunning and angelic one!) who now had to become the priority.

The point I wish to make here is that now that I have done my own RESET, and brought my Primary and Secondary Foods into comfortable alliance with each other, not only am I happier, but I am able to give stronger support and guidance to my husband and my family in ways I hadn't thought possible before.

And so if one of your goals is to achieve and maintain weight loss, just know that you must continually strive to improve the balance between your Primary and Secondary foods. The more balance achieved between these foods, the closer you are to Optimal Health, and to creating the space necessary to achieve your weight loss goals as well as other personal and professional goals.

Will it happen overnight? Perhaps not. Will we falter and sometimes fall? But of course. But the joy of the journey is picking ourselves back up and to keep moving FORWARD. We do the best we can with each and every passing day because we know once it's gone we never get it back. And we make the small incremental changes to our lifestyle as described here, and then hold ourselves accountable to the change!

I hope you take this opportunity to embrace the journey and to join the Lean Clean Movement, because if you do, I truly believe that the very best is yet to come!